MEOWGA

I0105855

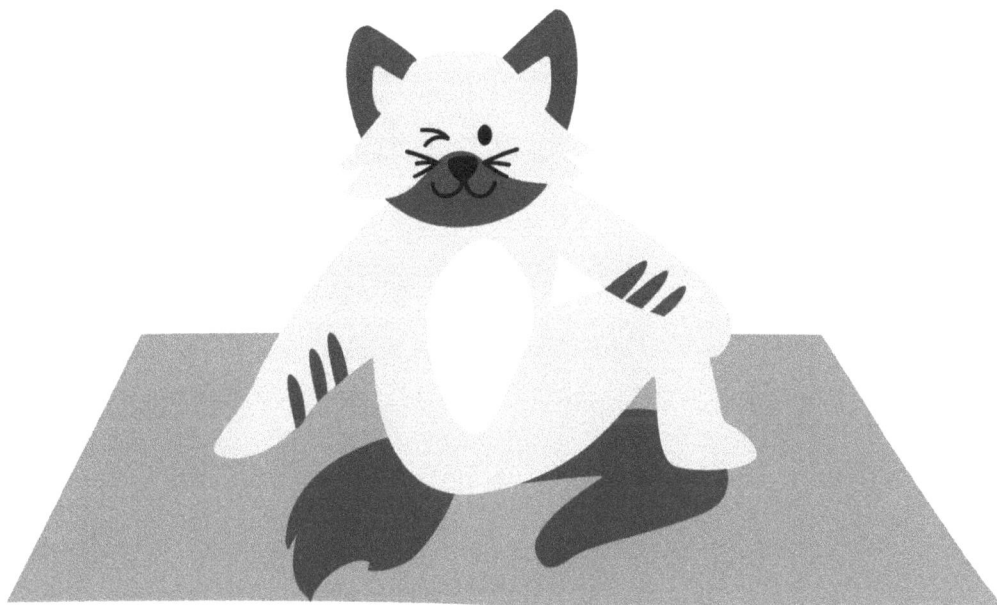

BY LIZ PALMIERI-COONLEY

MEOWGA

ISBN-13: 978-1-949142-02-0

Printed in the United States of America

MAY THE ENTIRE UNIVERSE BE FILLED WITH PEACE AND JOY, LOVE AND LIGHT.

MAY ALL BEINGS EVERYWHERE BE HAPPY AND FREE.

IN SOME WAY, MAY I CONTRIBUTE TO THAT HAPPINESS AND FREEDOM FOR ALL.

WITH LOVE & GRATITUDE,

LIZ

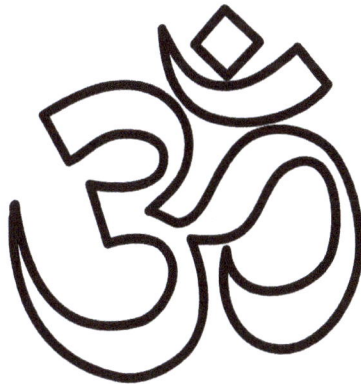

CRESCENT MOON

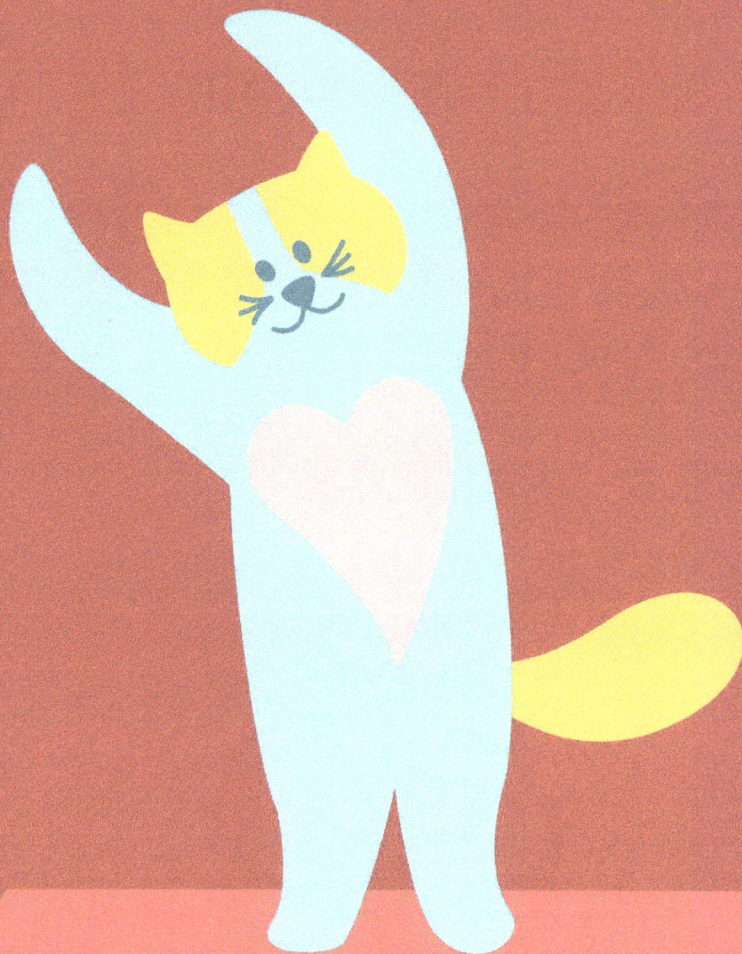

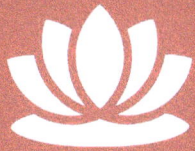

STAND WITH FEET TOGETHER

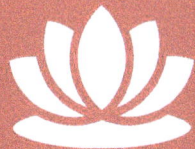

RAISE ARMS TO THE SKY

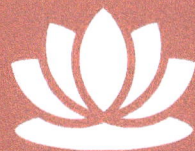

BEND TO THE LEFT & THEN BEND TO THE RIGHT

STRADDLE

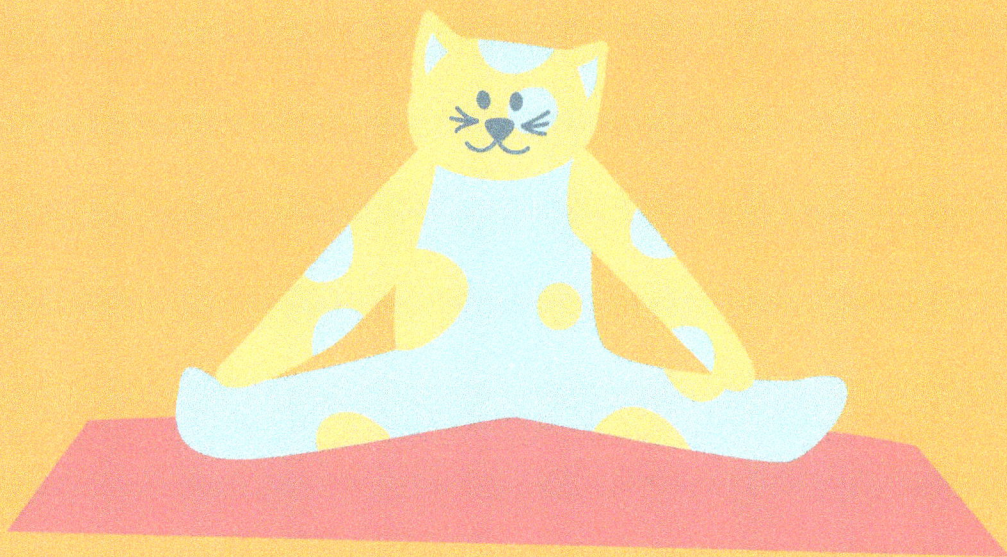

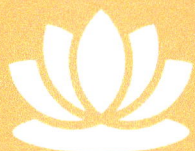

SIT WITH LEGS OUT IN FRONT OF YOU

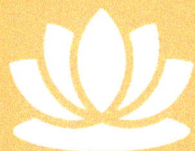

POINT LEFT FOOT LEFT & RIGHT FOOT RIGHT

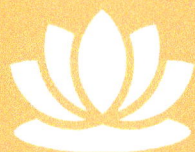

WALK YOUR HANDS OUT IN FRONT OF YOU

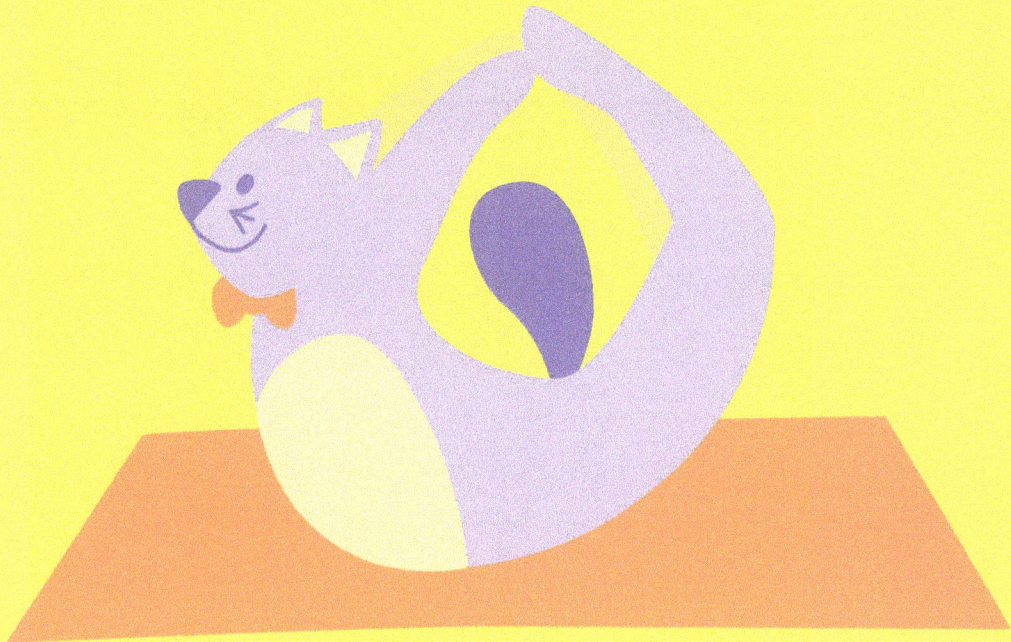

BOW

SPINE TWIST

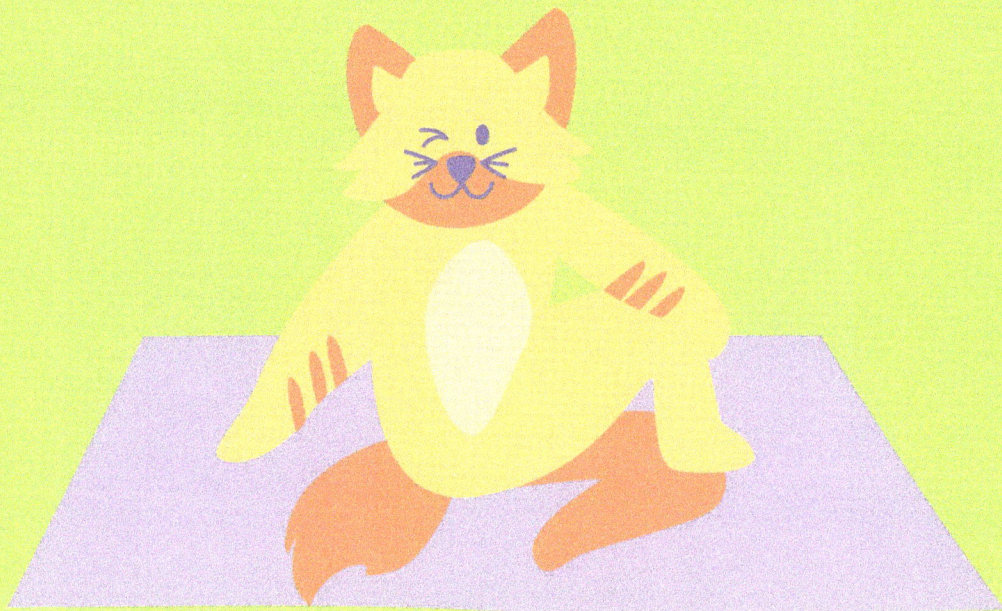

SIT CRISSCROSS
APPLESAUCE

PLACE ONE HAND ON
OPPOSITE KNEE AND
THE OTHER HAND
BEHIND YOU

UNPRETZEL YOUR
LEGS & REPEAT ON
THE OTHER SIDE

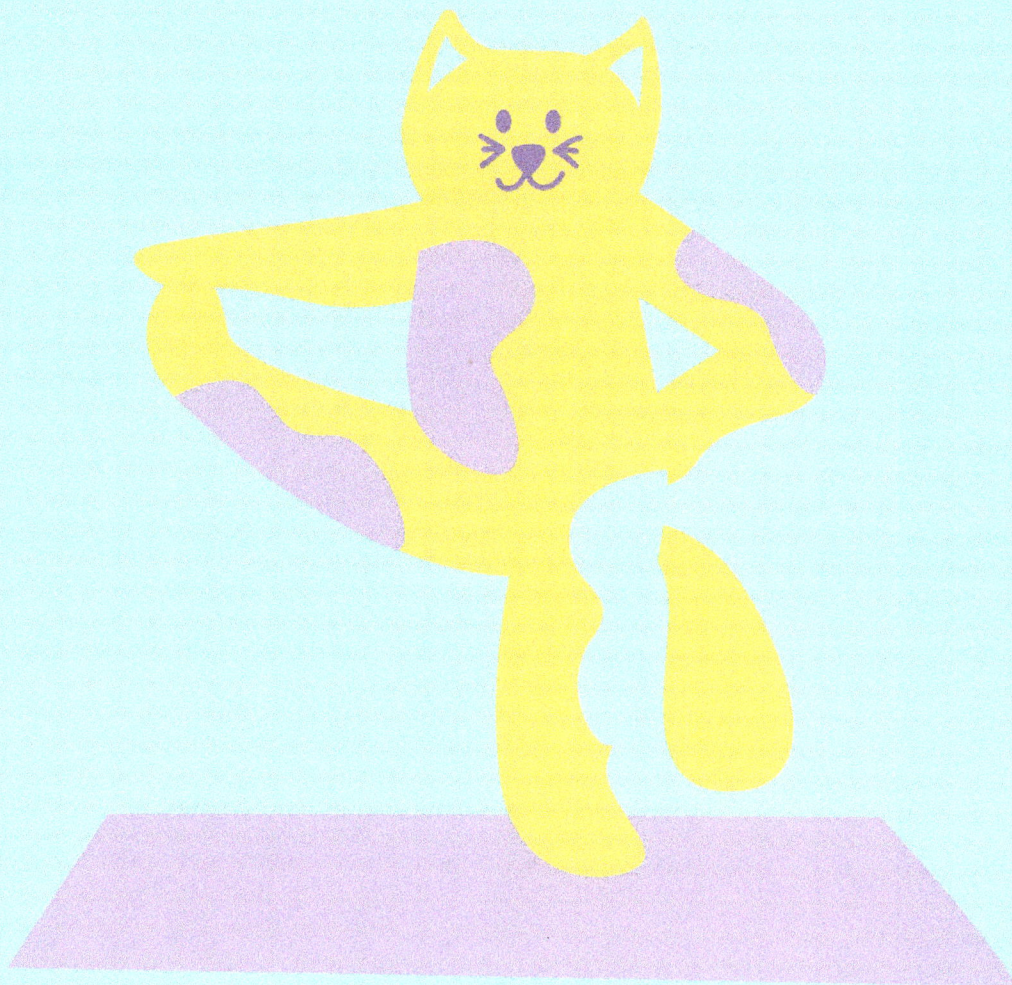

BIG TOE

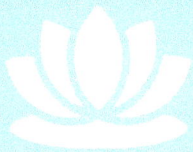

STAND WITH FEET
TOGETHER

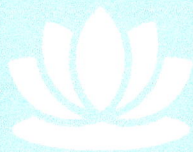

SLOWLY BEND ONE
KNEE & BALANCE ON
ONE FOOT

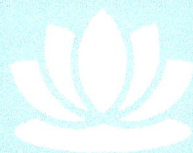

GRAB YOUR BIG TOE
& EXTEND LEG OUT
TO THE SIDE

STAR

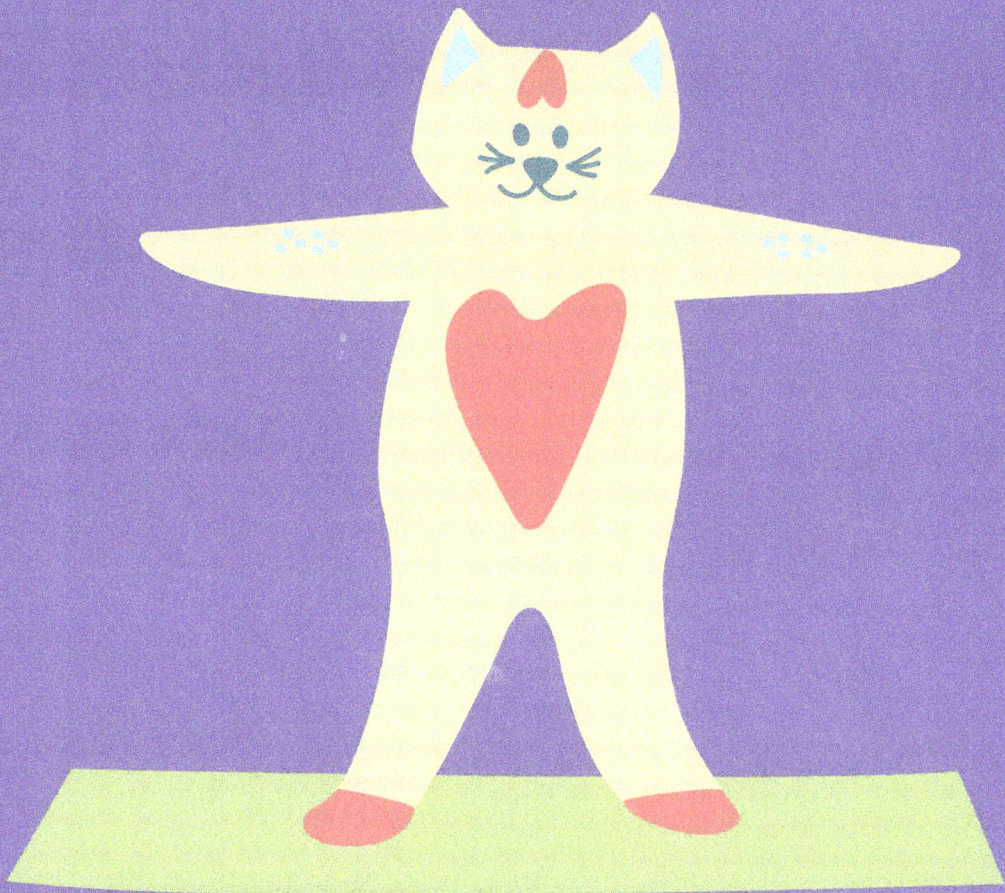

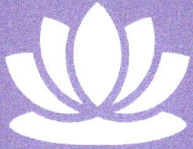

STAND WITH FEET APART

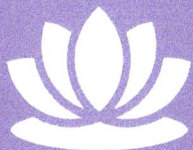

REACH ARMS OUT WIDE

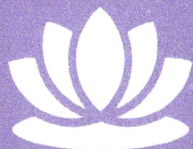

SMILE BIG & SAY "I'M A STAR!"

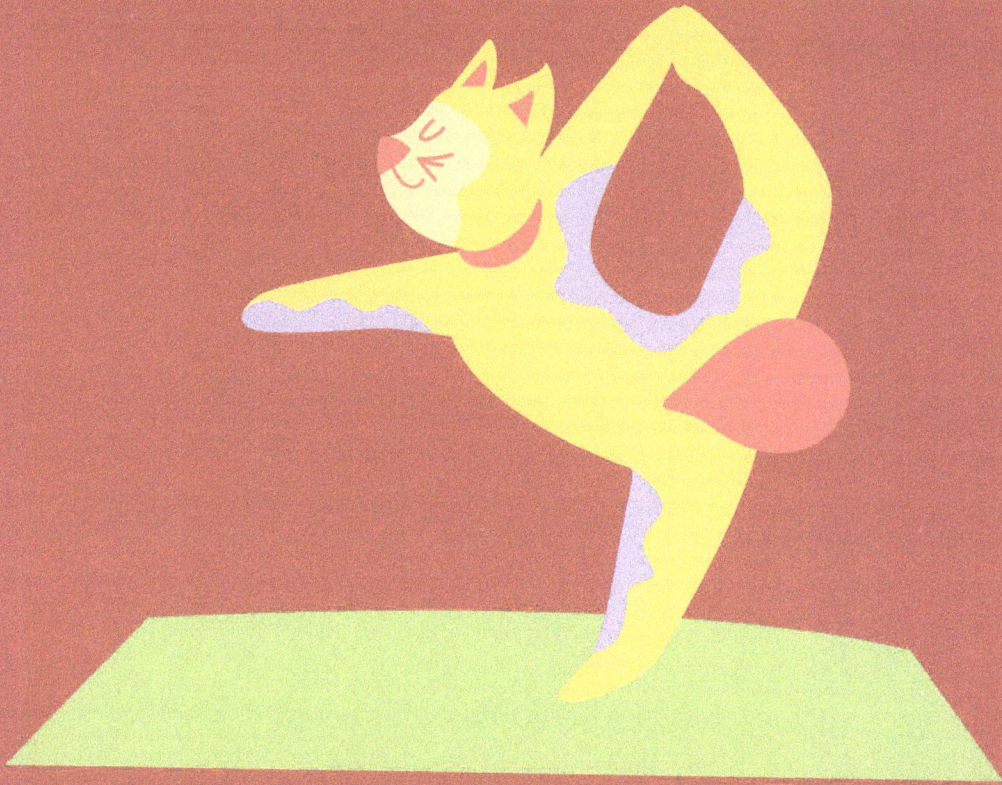

DANCER

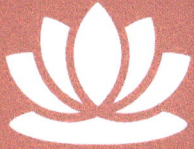

STAND WITH FEET TOGETHER

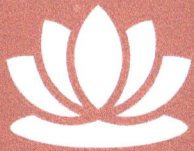

SLOWLY BEND ONE KNEE & BALANCE ON ONE FOOT

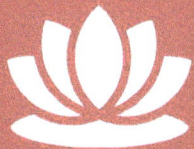

REACH BEHIND YOU & GRAB THE ANKLE OF THE RAISED KNEE

UP DOG

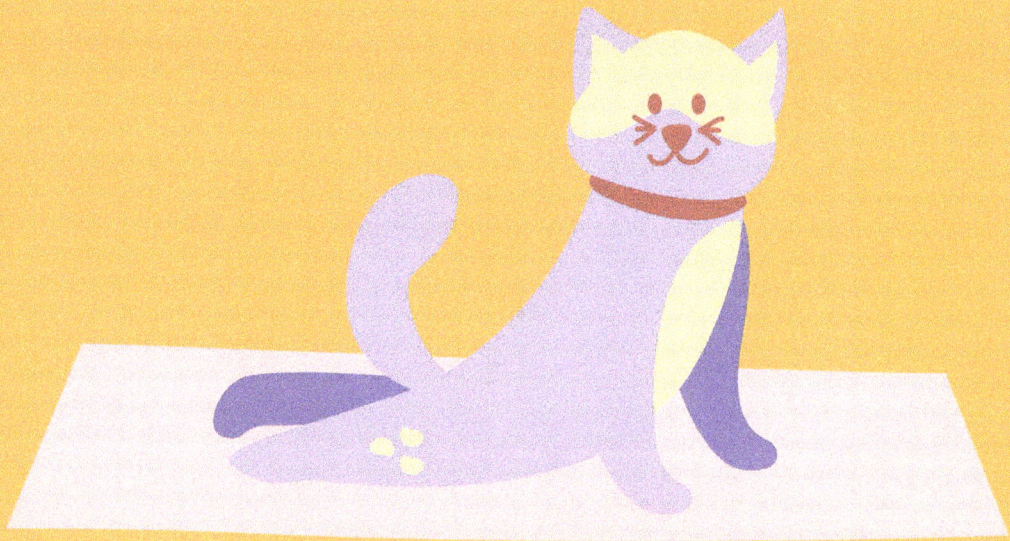

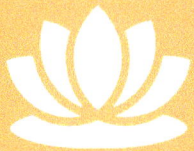

LAY ON YOUR BELLY

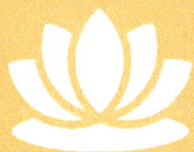

PLANT HANDS UNDER
SHOULDERS

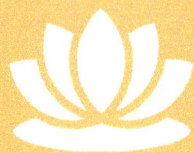

STRAIGHTEN ARMS
AND LIFT HEAD

TREE

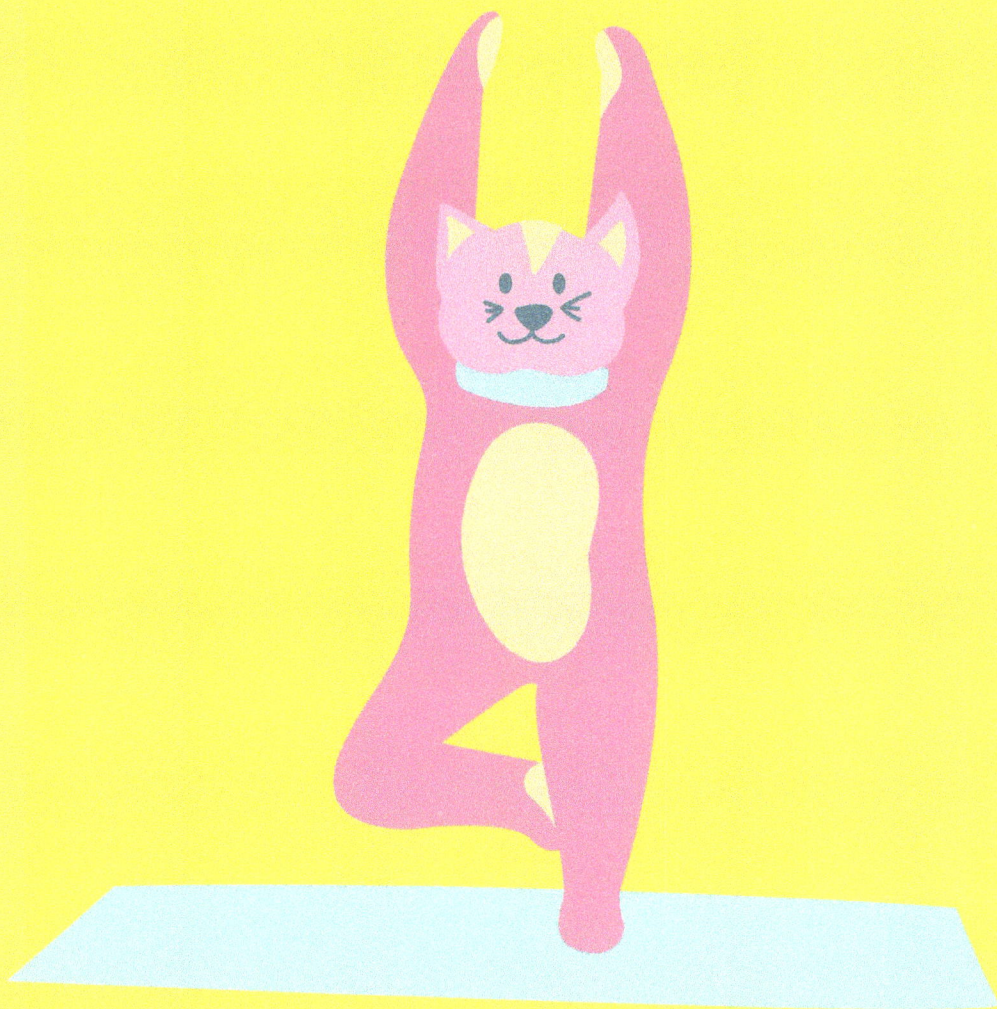

SHOULDER STAND

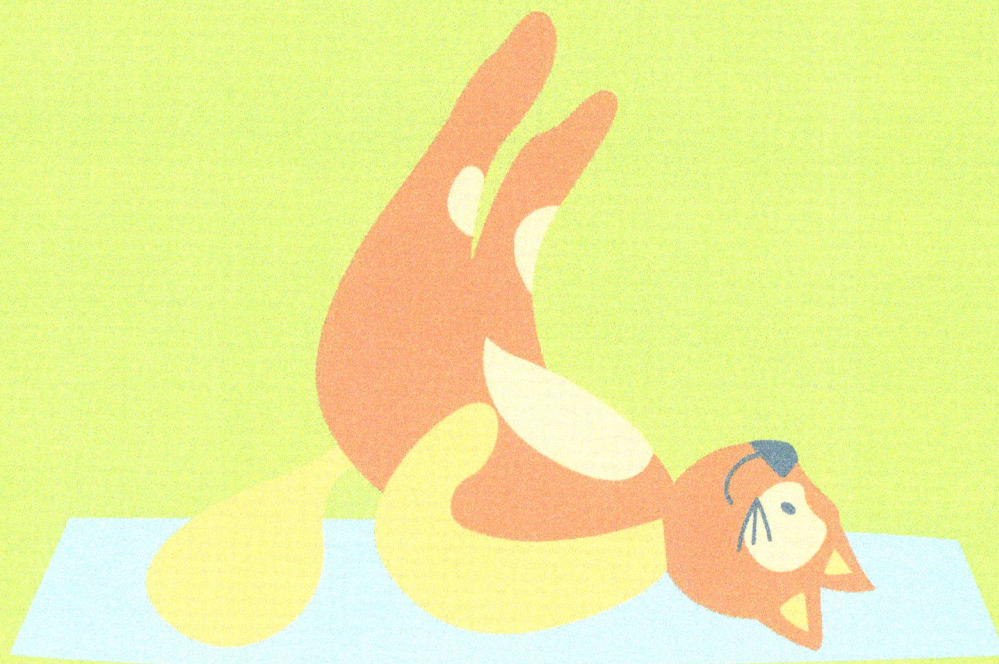

LAY ON YOUR BACK

LIFT YOUR LEGS
TOWARDS THE SKY

PUT YOUR HANDS ON
YOUR LOW BACK TO
HELP RAISE LEGS

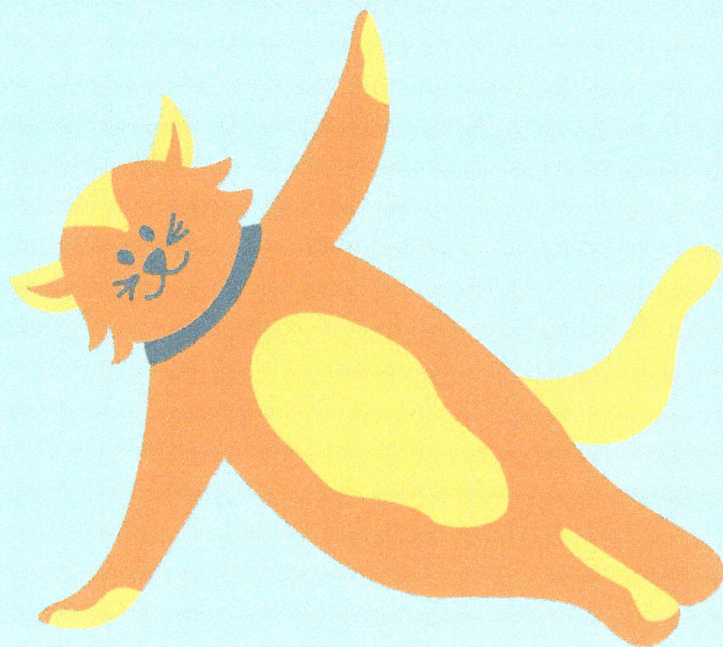

SIDE PLANK

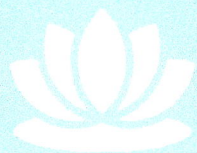

GET ON ALL FOURS

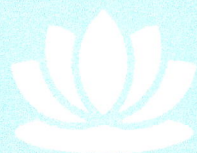

SHIFT ALL YOUR WEIGHT TO THE LEFT ARM & LEFT LEG

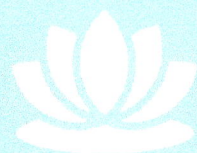

PUSH AWAY FROM FLOOR WITH HAND & FOOT

WARRIOR I

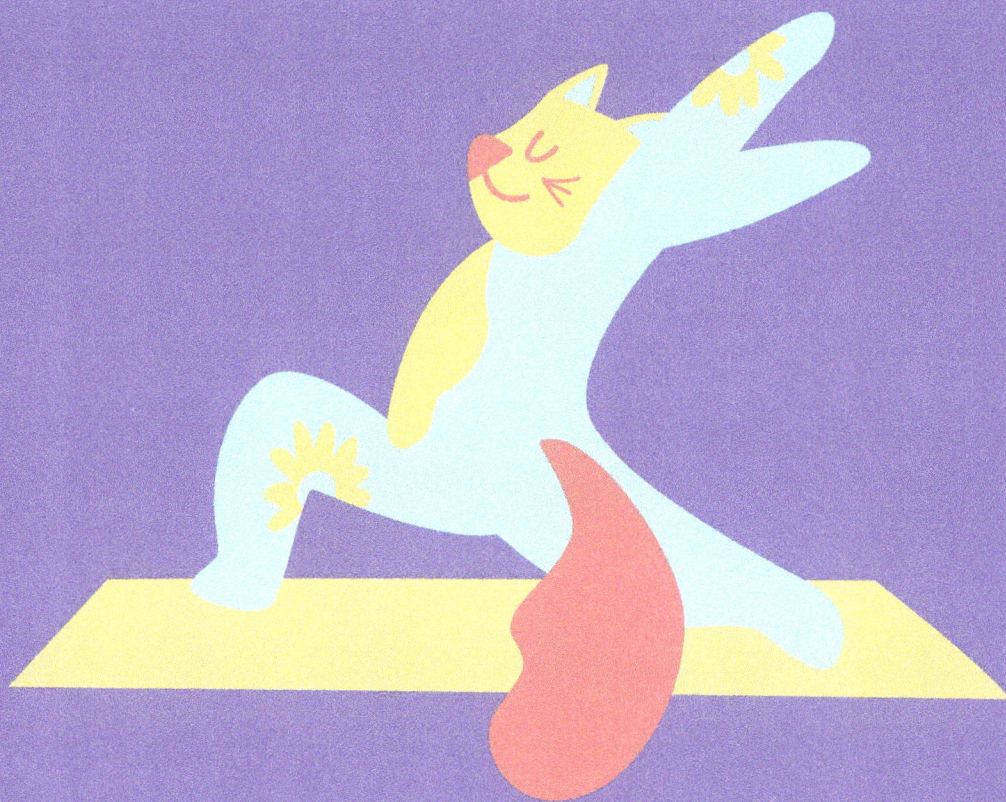

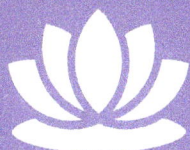

BEND FRONT KNEE

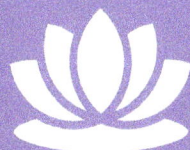

POINT BACK FOOT
AWAY FROM BODY

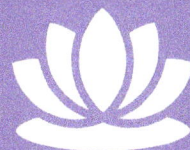

RAISE ARMS TO THE
SKY

SIDE STRETCH

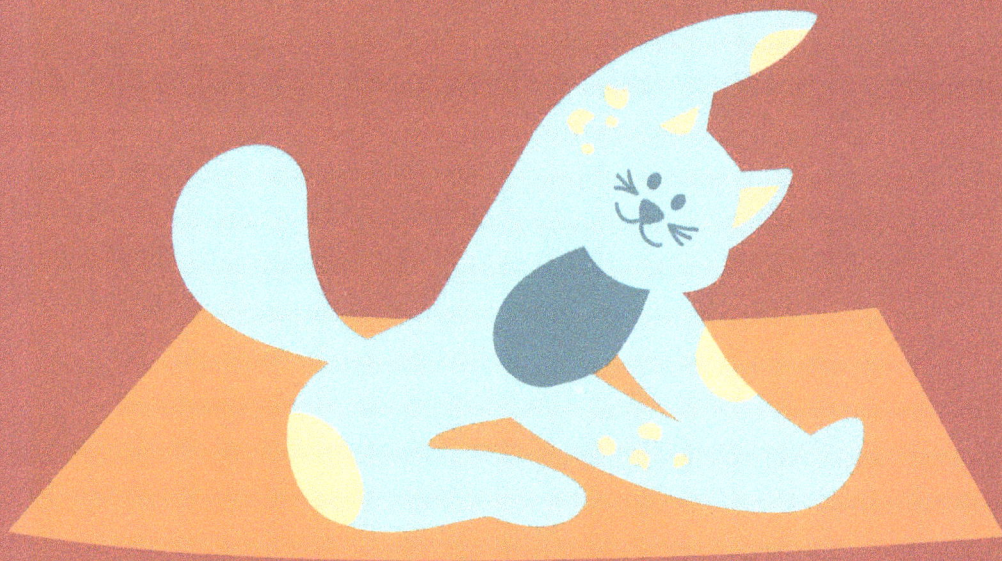

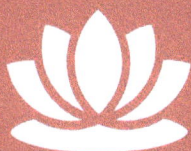

SIT WITH LEGS OUT
IN FRONT OF YOU

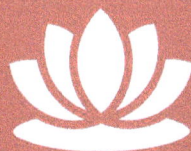

BRING LEFT FOOT
INSIDE RIGHT THIGH

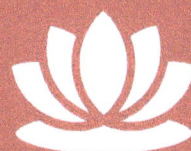

RAISE LEFT ARM TO
SKY & LEAN TO THE
RIGHT

WARRIOR 2

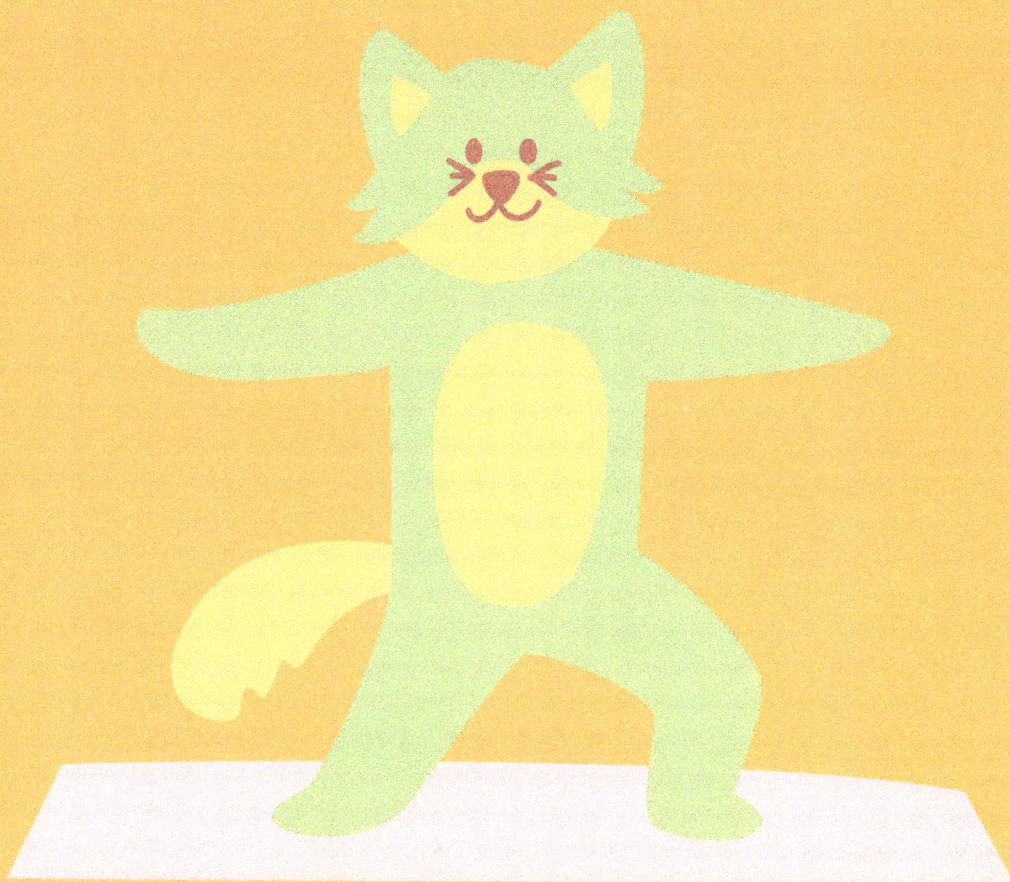

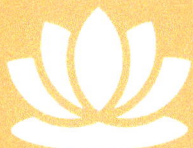

BEND FRONT KNEE

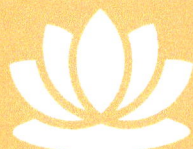

POINT BACK FOOT
TO THE SIDE

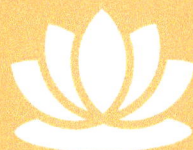

STRETCH ARMS OUT
WIDE

BOAT

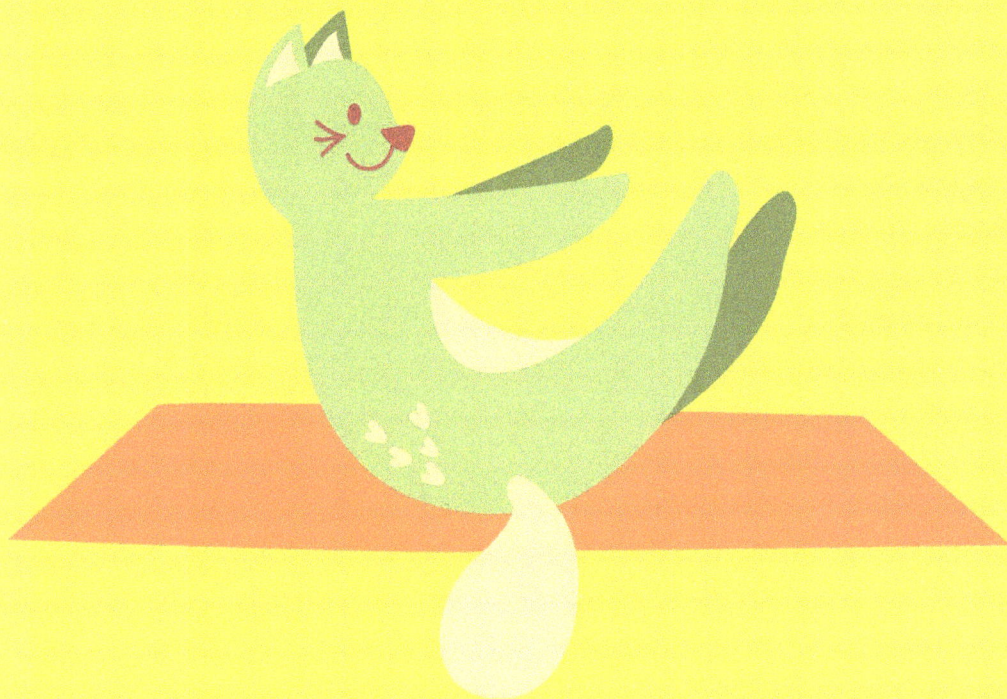

SUNBIRD

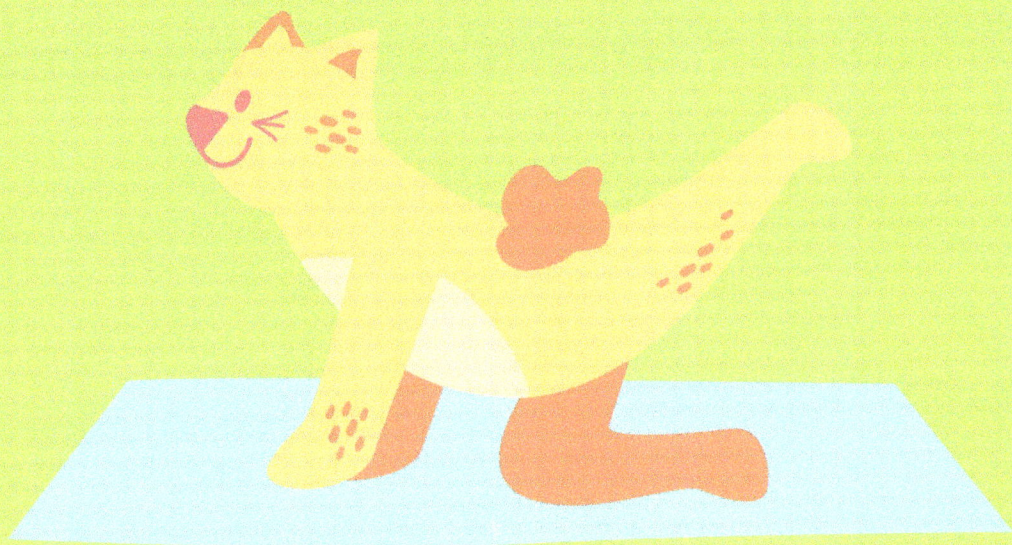

GET ON ALL FOURS

STRETCH OUT YOUR
RIGHT ARM & LEFT
LEG

REPEAT ON THE
OTHER SIDE

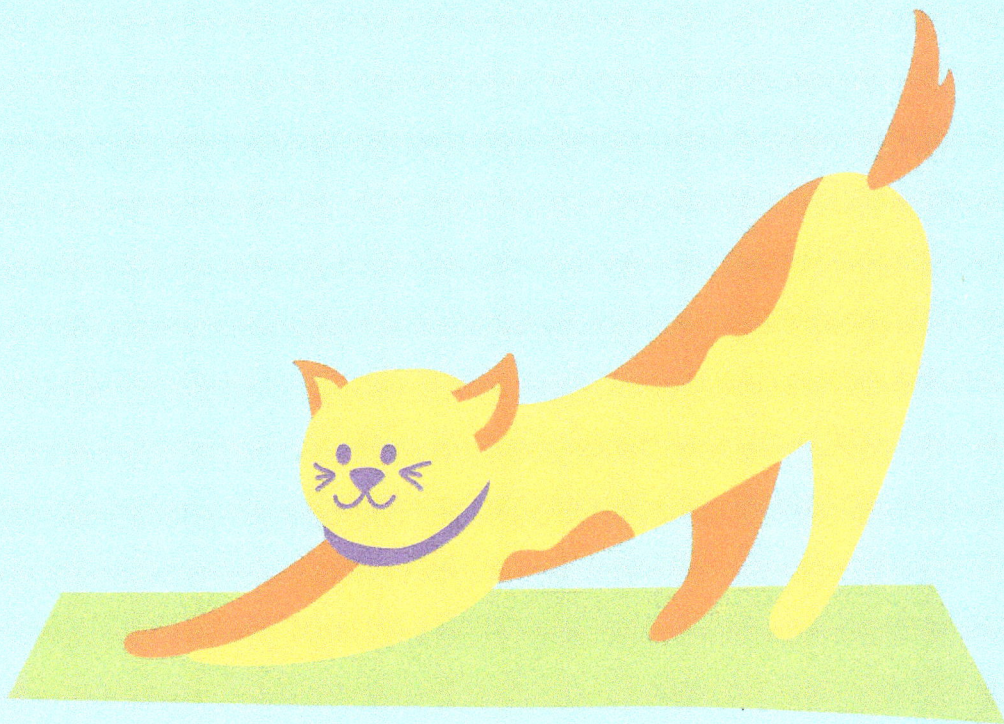

DOWN DOG

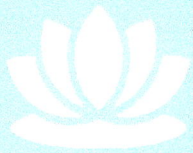

GET ON ALL FOURS
& STRAIGHTEN KNEES

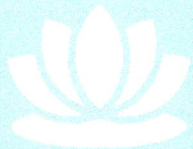

TUSHY TOWARDS THE
SKY

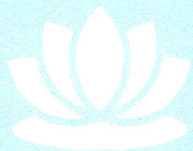

HEAD BETWEEN ARMS

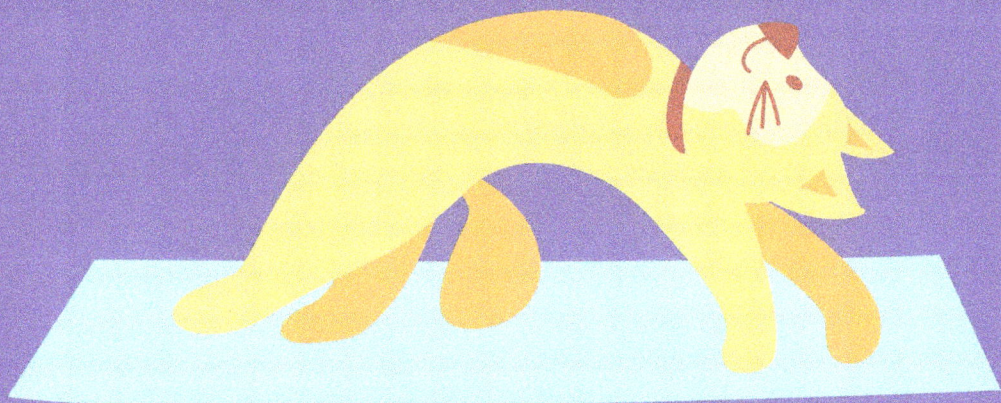

WHEEL

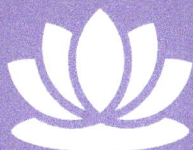

LAY ON YOUR BACK

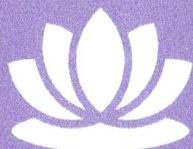

PLANT YOUR HANDS
& FEET ON THE
FLOOR

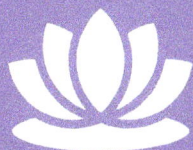

ADULT LIFTS YOUR
BACK AS YOU PUSH
AWAY FROM FLOOR

COW FACE

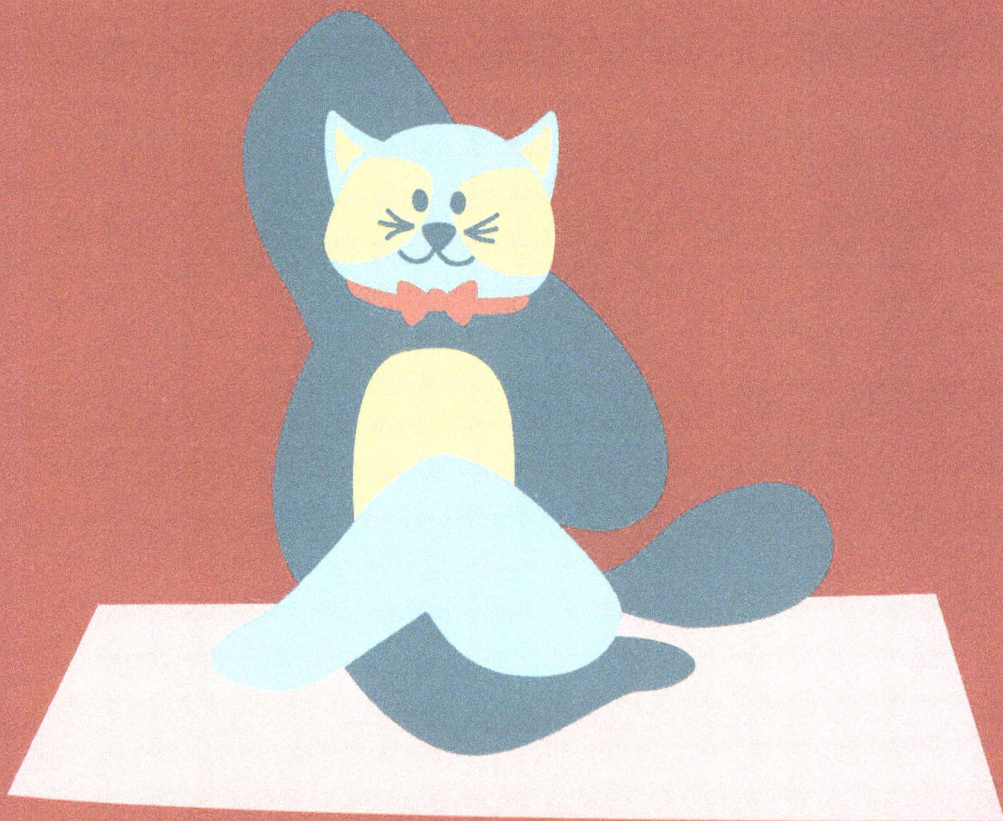

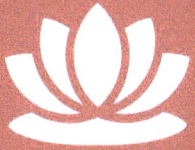

SIT WITH LEGS OUT
IN FRONT OF YOU

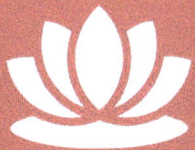

MOVE LEFT FOOT
UNDER RIGHT
TOWARDS TUSHY

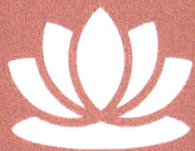

STACK RIGHT LEG ON
TOP WITH LEFT FOOT
TOWARDS TUSHY

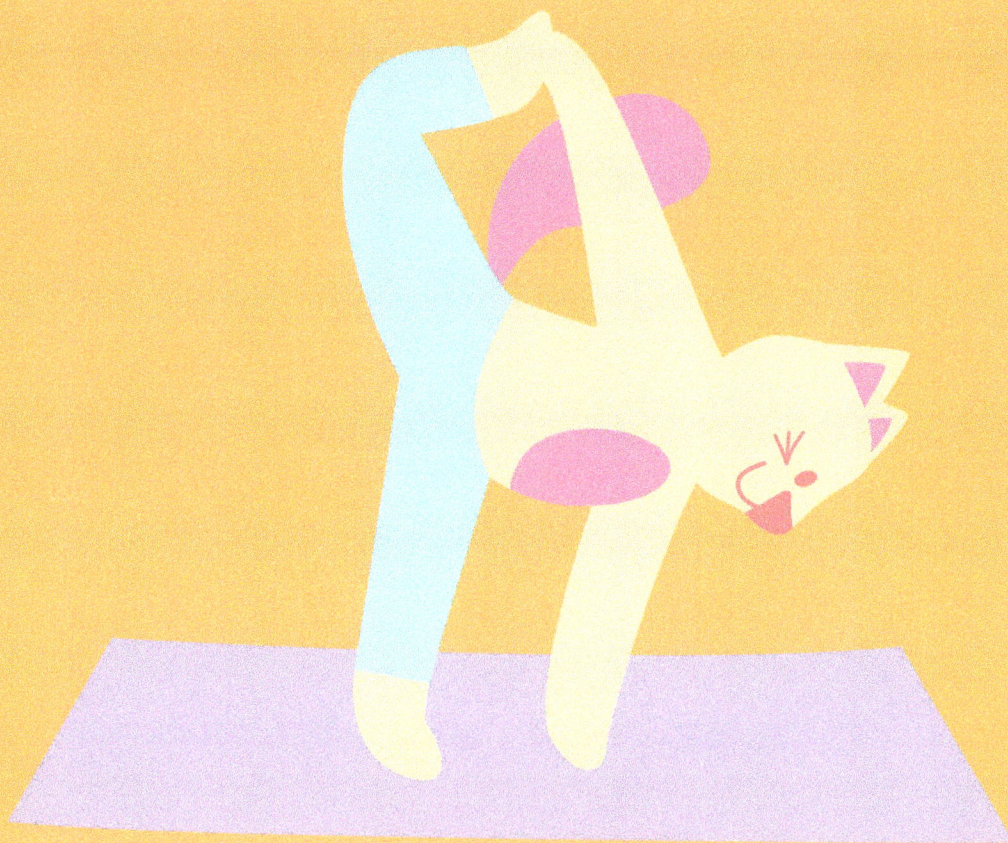

HALF MOON

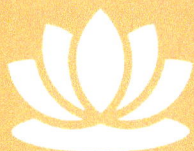

STAND WITH FEET TOGETHER

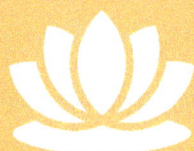

PLACE LEFT HAND DOWN ON THE GROUND

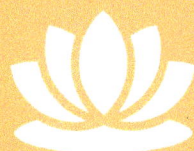

SLOWLY RAISE RIGHT LEG OFF OF THE GROUND

MOUNTAIN

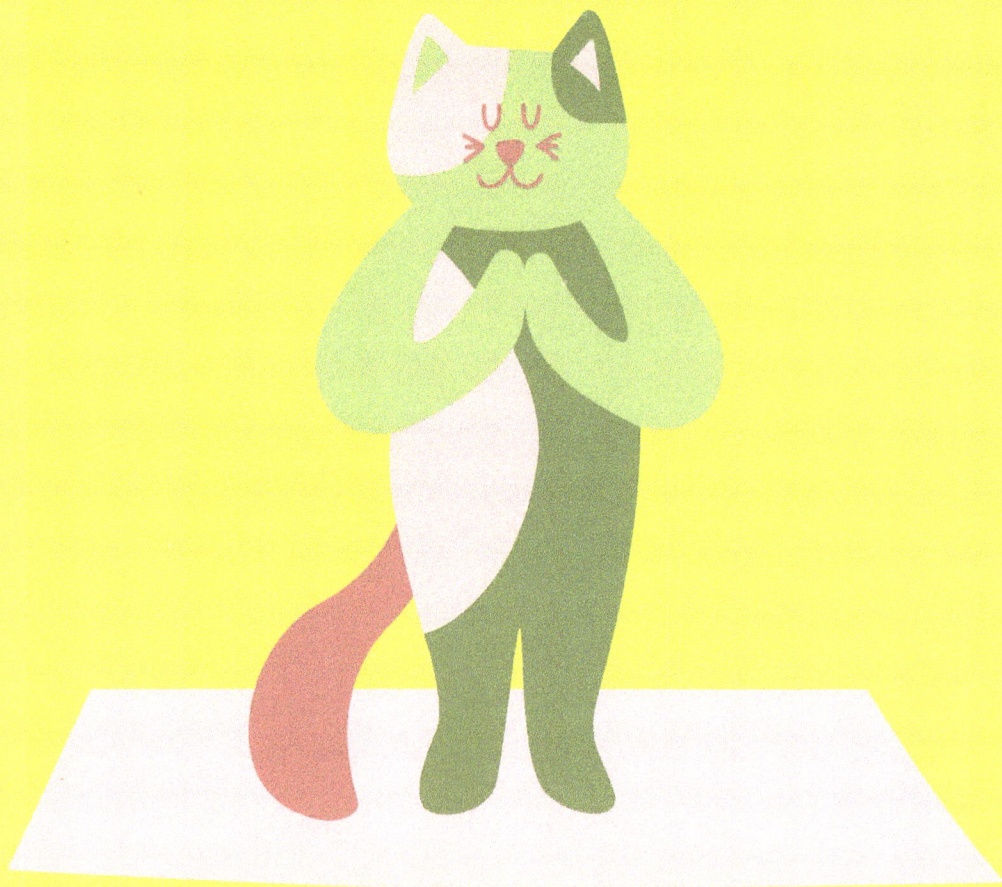

HANDSTAND

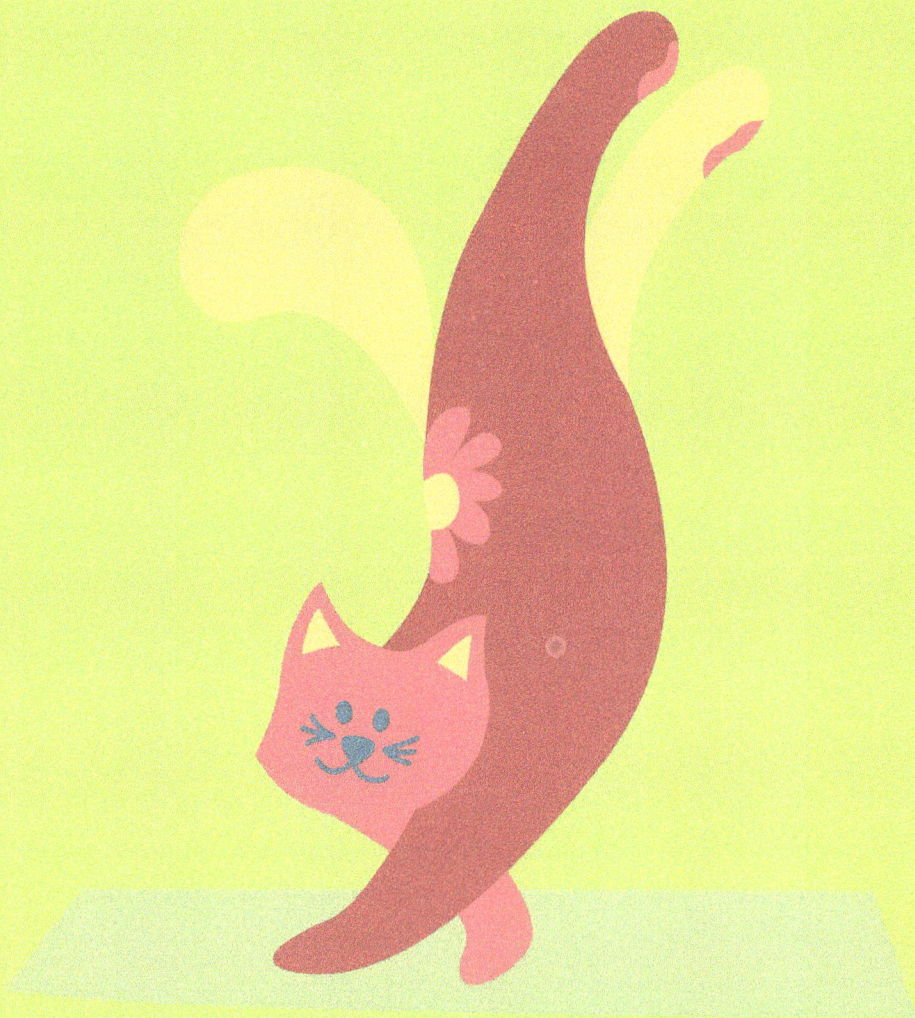

LAY ON BELLY

HAVE AN ADULT LIFT
YOU UP BY YOUR
ANKLES

PLANT YOUR HANDS
ON THE GROUND &
STRAIGHTEN ARMS

LOW LUNGE

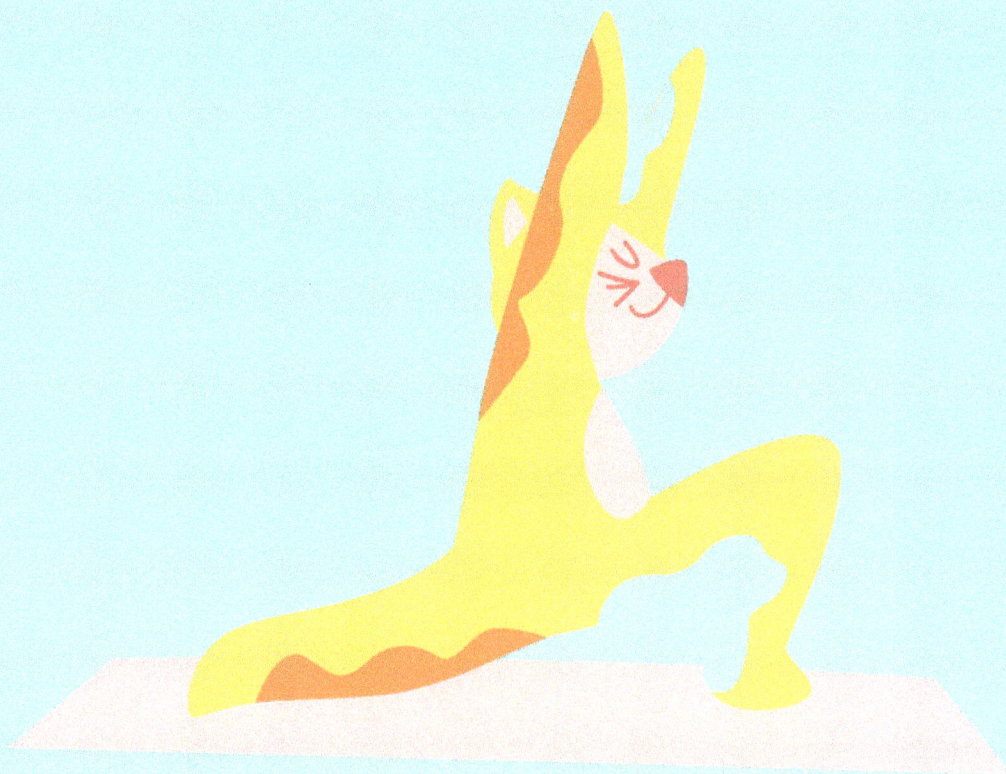

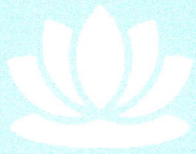

GET ON ALL FOURS

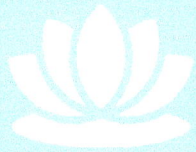

STEP ONE FOOT FORWARD

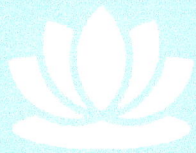

RAISE ARMS TO THE SKY

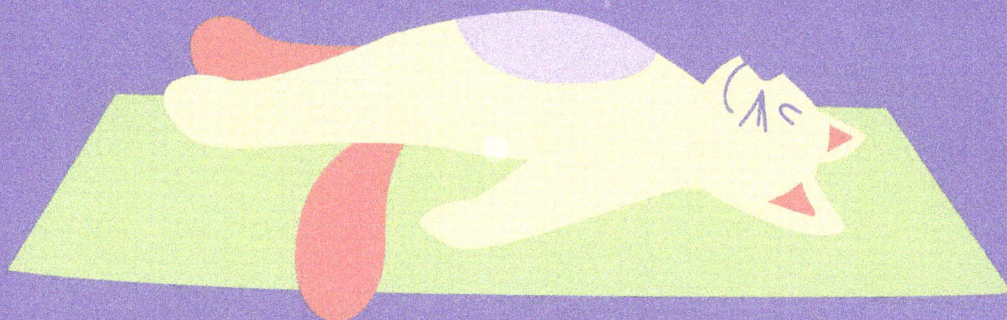

BEDTIME

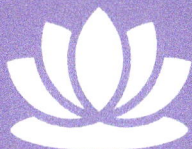

LAY ON YOUR BACK

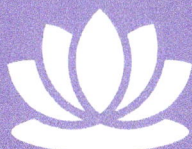

GET AS
COMFORTABLE AS
POSSIBLE

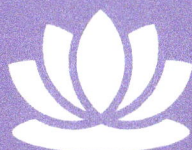

CLOSE YOUR EYES
AND SMILE

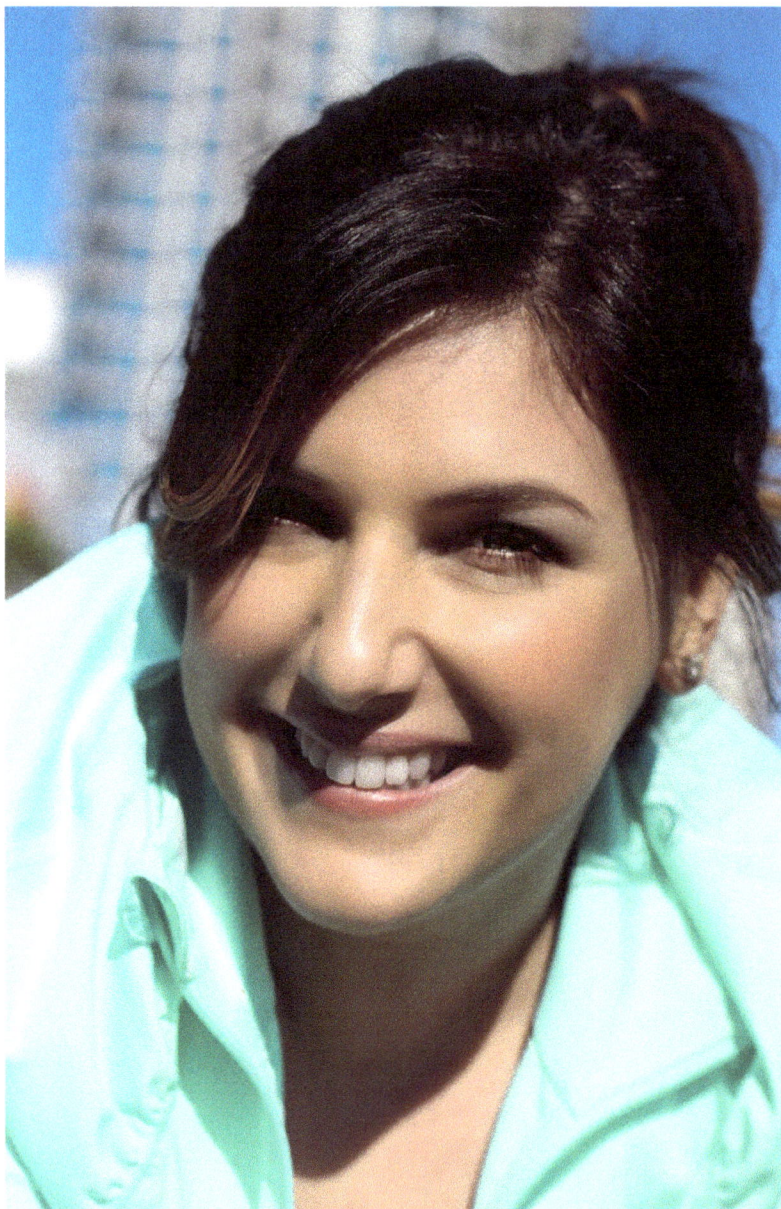

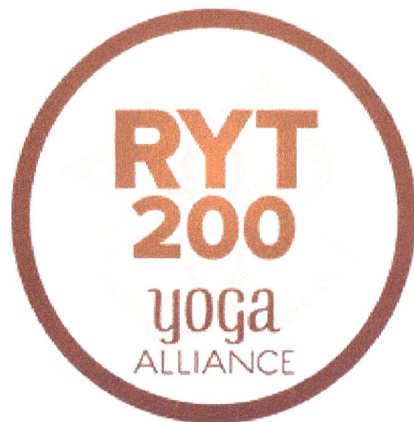

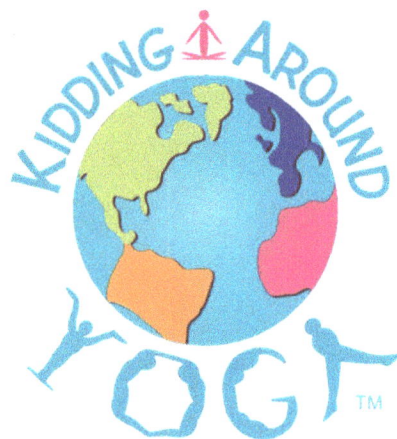

ABOUT THE AUTHOR

Liz Palmieri-Coonley is an author, 200-hour Registered Yoga Teacher, and Integrative Nutrition Health Coach. She is also a Certified Kids Yoga Teacher with Kidding Around Yoga.

She grew up with a fascination for the human body, illness, and healing, which may seem weird for a kid, but it makes total sense considering both of her parents were in the medical field.

In addition to her love for educating others on yoga and holistic health, Liz is passionate about traveling, spending time outdoors, and everything about her incredible nieces. Some of her more epic adventures include: scuba diving, climbing a waterfall, and riding in a hot air balloon.

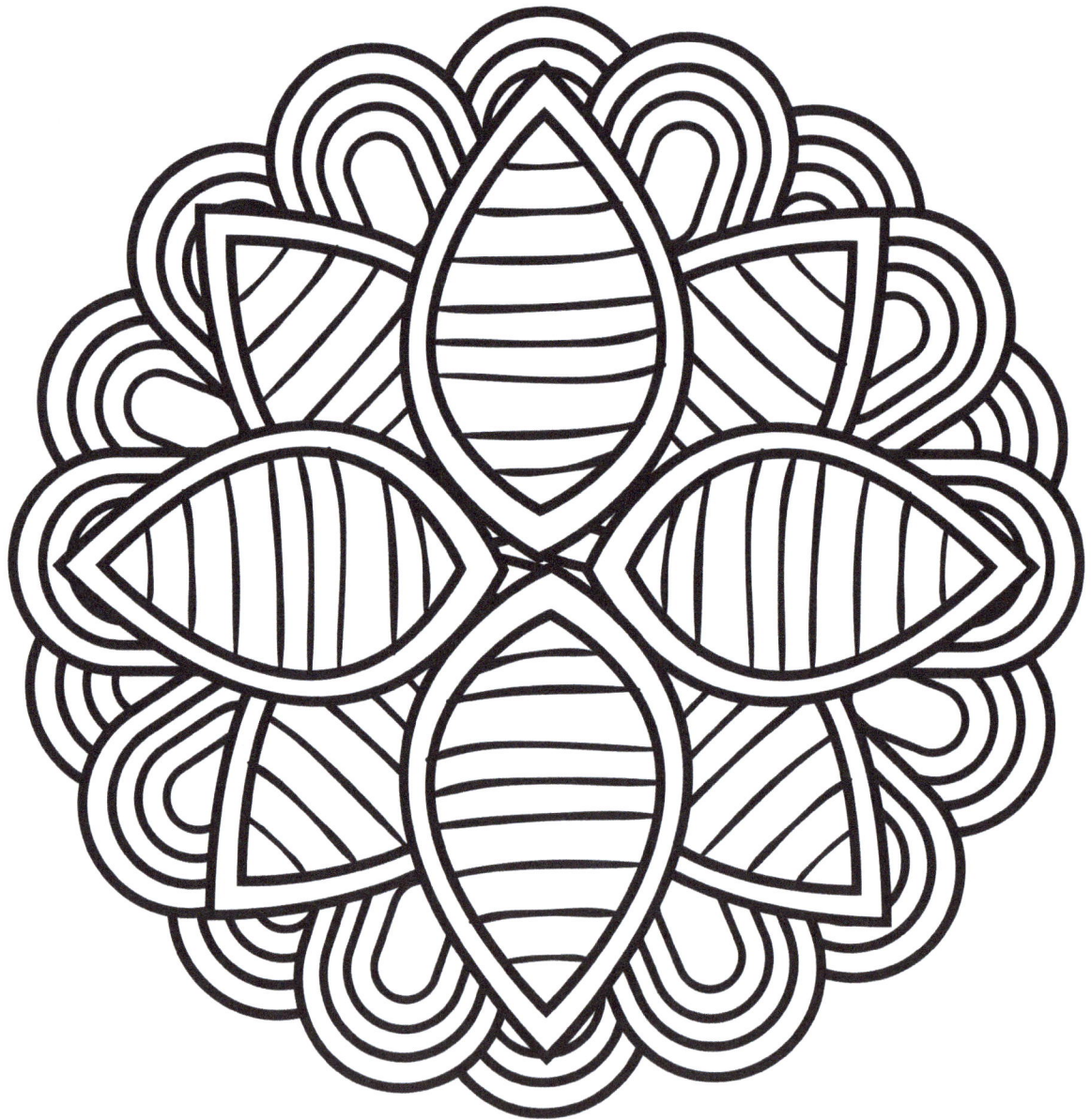

www.ingramcontent.com/pod-product-compliance
Lightning Source LLC
Chambersburg PA
CBHW042333030426

42335CB00027B/3322